THE FARMER GYM WAY

HYBRID TRAINING FOR MAXIMIZING FITNESS

THE FARMER GYM WAY
HYBRID TRAINING FOR MAXIMIZING FITNESS

The Farmer Gym Way is a 14-week strength, conditioning, and cardio program designed to improve one's strength and overall fitness level. With heavy-weight lifting, high-intensity interval training, and endurance-based training, the program challenges the whole body, both anaerobically and aerobically. The Farmer Gym Way anticipates that you will work out 4 days a week, with 2 days of built-in rest, and a day of running once each week – except for the 3 deload weeks and 2 testing weeks. You will proceed through the program day by day, just as you would a daily calendar.

The training structure is simple. Each primary workout begins with a "strength" portion, consisting of the Deadlift, Squat, Bench Press, or Overhead Press. The particular strength exercise should be executed for the stated number of sets and repetitions. For example: Week 2, Day 1 consists of the Deadlift; for this session, you will perform 3 sets, at 8 repetitions per set, based on 70-75% of your 1 Repetition Max (1RM). The percentage range allows you to autoregulate your lift: if 70% feels light, go with a higher percentage; if it feels too heavy, lower the weight. Rest between each set should last at least 2 minutes. Give yourself enough time to recover, but not so much time that you cool off. Each primary workout finishes with a "conditioning" segment, consisting of high-intensity interval training and/or endurance-based training. Although each conditioning workout is randomized and unique, each is intended to complement the strength portion of that day's workout. You should perform all the movements in the manner presented in the next section of this book.

Built into the conditioning portion of The Farmer Gym Way are mechanisms for making the workouts more or less challenging. You can increase the weight as you become stronger. You can increase or decrease the amount of rest as you move through the workout. Don't be afraid to kick up the intensity if you find that you aren't breathing heavily or feeling some exhaustion during the workouts. But, take as many seconds of rest as you need during these workouts in order to safely perform the remainder of a set or the next round. Your goal should be to work out for the entire duration of each workout, even if that means taking longer rests between sets. Never push yourself beyond your limits at the expense of good form or breathing. It's always better to take a break and recover than to burn out and quit or to lose your form and injure yourself.

Each workout in the program includes its own notes section, where you can jot down your performance, measure your progress, and note any adjustments. This will serve to help you not only learn about your body, but also be encouraged as you see your performance improve on the various workouts. If competition motivates you, then make it a competition against yourself (or a friend!), and keep score. For example: if on Week 2, Day 2 you perform your conditioning in 35:21, write it down. When you come back to this workout later in the program, during Week 6 or Week 10, attempt to better your performance by completing the workout faster (without sacrificing form). The competition aspect also applies to week-to-week strength gains, as you monitor your progress.

At the beginning and end of the 14 weeks are a "testing" segment, consisting of 16 parameters of fitness, challenging your strength, strength-endurance, and endurance. These parameters are set in place to measure enhancements in performance. We hope and believe that after you navigate through the 3 months of work, your overall fitness will have improved.

WHO IS THE FARMER GYM WAY FOR?

This book is not for beginners; we recommend you have at least a year's worth of experience in the weight room and with high-intensity interval training before using the program. Most of the exercises found here should be familiar to you; if they aren't, we recommend becoming proficient in them before proceeding. This book is not for advanced weightlifters. (We don't wish to discourage elite lifters from using the program--we simply want to emphasize the fact that this group of individuals utilizes a very regimented programming scheme, one specifically designed to strictly increase strength.) The Farmer Gym Way is for those with weightlifting experience who wish to increase strength and overall fitness by challenging their personal bests and testing their physical limits. If you are searching for the "bulky" look, or a "skinny" frame, this book is also not for you; designed to grow strong, healthy, long-lasting muscle, this program is geared toward an "athletic" look.

THE EQUIPMENT

To use The Farmer Gym Way, you'll need access to a gym, or to have several pieces of equipment at your disposal. The equipment: Barbell and accompanying weight, Dumbbells, Kettlebell, Pull-up Bar, Dip Box/Bars, Box, Jump Rope, Rower, Treadmill/Track. These tools are great for building strength, power, stability, and cardiovascular endurance. Found in gyms everywhere, the Barbell and Dumbbell are popular weight-bearing pieces that require the body to generate power, thus developing one's strength. The Kettlebell, a more novel piece of equipment, requires the body to exert force and maintain balance in a number of positions, due to its weight and changing center of gravity during use. The ever popular Pull-up Bar and Dip Bars are body-weight apparatuses, designed for lifting and moving oneself through a range of motion for muscle production. The Jump Rope, Box, Rower, Stationary Bike, and Treadmill/Track (or just some place to run) are specifically geared for muscular endurance and building stamina. Your gym *should* have these.

THE STRENGTH WORKOUTS

The strength workouts in this program are to be executed for a specific number of sets and repetitions for a particular percentage range of your 1RM. If you don't know your 1RM, you will need to test your lift. The sets and reps should be difficult but not impossible. If you're able to easily handle the repetitions, especially on the last set, increasing the weight is advised. It's important to use a spotter during this portion of the workout, or otherwise when necessary—in particular, for the Squat and Bench Press; you will not need a spot for the Deadlift. Another thing to keep in mind: rest. Be certain to recoup between sets, resting at least 2 minutes before proceeding to the next round of work. This kind of heavy-weight training has been found to improve muscular strength, increase bone mass, and elevate fat burning. The workouts are designed to use a high amount of weight over the set-rep combination (total volume) to help strengthen and shape the muscle.

HOW TO FIND YOUR 1RM

Your 1RM, the heaviest amount of weight you can lift once, is one of the truest measures of absolute strength. Using this information, a strength program can be effectively planned and executed.

There are two primary methods by which to test your 1RM: For those who have vast experience lifting, you'll begin with a proper warm-up and then gradually work your way up to a max-weight lift. For those who have little experience with max-weight testing, you will warm up, gradually work up in weight, and then take a number of reps at a specific weight and compare it to a corresponding percentage. For example, properly executing a lift for eight repetitions (you should not be able to lift the weight for a ninth rep) at 160 lbs. results in an *approximate* 80% 1RM, or a 200 lb. max lift. (See the chart below for more percentages.) Keep in mind, this is just an estimate, and the lower the number of reps you test, the more accurate you'll be.

When performing either of these methods, it's important to warm up first, progressively work up in weight, and use a spotter.

100%	95%	92.5%	90%	87.5%	85%	82.5%	80%	77.5%
1RM	2RM	3RM	4RM	5RM	6RM	7RM	8RM	9RM
100	95	92	90	87	85	82	80	77
105	99	97	94	91	89	86	84	81
110	104	101	99	96	93	90	88	85
115	109	106	103	100	97	94	92	89
120	114	111	108	105	102	99	96	93
125	118	115	112	19	106	103	100	96
130	123	120	117	113	110	107	104	100
135	128	124	121	118	114	111	108	104
140	133	129	126	122	119	115	112	108
145	137	134	130	126	123	119	116	112
150	142	138	135	131	127	123	120	116
155	147	143	139	135	131	127	124	120
160	152	148	144	140	136	132	128	124
165	156	152	148	144	140	136	132	127
170	161	157	153	148	144	140	136	131
175	166	161	157	153	148	144	140	135
180	171	166	162	157	153	148	144	139
185	175	171	166	161	157	152	148	143
190	180	175	171	166	161	156	152	147
195	185	180	175	170	165	160	156	151
200	190	185	180	175	170	165	160	155
205	194	189	184	179	174	169	164	158
210	199	194	189	183	178	173	168	162
215	204	198	193	188	182	177	172	166
220	209	203	195	192	187	181	176	170
225	213	208	202	196	191	185	180	174
230	218	212	207	201	195	189	184	178
235	223	217	211	205	199	193	188	182
240	228	222	216	210	204	198	192	186
245	232	226	220	214	208	202	196	189
250	237	231	225	218	212	206	200	193

*Additional charts with expanded numbers can be found online.

THE CONDITIONING WORKOUTS

The conditioning workouts are designed to test various areas of fitness, and they range in duration. Although many workouts will last for 30 minutes or more, several do not. This might make you skeptical. But research has shown that vigorous exercise sessions lasting for relatively short periods of time are very effective in achieving fitness results. This kind of high-intensity workout has been found to improve cardiovascular health, increase lean muscle, elevate fat burning, and boost energy levels. And, because the workouts are designed to use a high number of repetitions to take the muscles near fatigue, these workouts tear down the muscle fibers, which can help lead to muscle toning and strengthening. So whether shorter or longer in duration, the goal is to push yourself and test your physical prowess.

Always be careful when selecting your equipment weight, and don't attempt to increase the weight too quickly. We have a recommended weight range for the various workouts, but you should start with lower weights and gradually increase the size of the weight you are using. It's important to perform each exercise correctly before moving up in weight. Some professionals recommend that females start with a weight between 10 and 20 pounds for Dumbbells and between 15 and 25 pounds for Kettlebells, gradually increasing in weight; it's recommended that males start with a weight between 15 and 30 pounds for Dumbbells and between 25 and 35 pounds for Kettlebells, gradually increasing in weight. If you can perform 15–20 repetitions without becoming fatigued, you may want to increase your weight. If you have several years of experience, you may be able to easily handle heavier weights. Know your limits, but remember: results begin at the edge of your comfort zone.

When choosing the correct box height for the conditioning workouts, err on the side of caution. Start with lower heights and gradually increase the height of the box. It's important to perform each jump correctly. If you feel nervous about using a box or are unable to, perform the Tuck Jump or Jumping Jack.

A WORD ON NUTRITION

A substantial part of health and wellness lies in proper nutrition. When an exercise regimen is adopted in conjunction with a healthful diet, the results are synergistic. Although nutrition is beyond the scope of this book, Farmer Gym emphatically encourages healthy eating to more effectively achieve your fitness goals. If you eat like garbage, your body will not respond to the workouts of this or any other program. (You can't outwork a bad diet!)

A WORD ON SLEEP

The best workout and a perfect diet cannot make up for insufficient sleep. Sleep is when muscle recovers; it's during sleep that growth-hormone production and protein synthesis help our muscles build. Our bodies benefit from 8 or more hours of sleep a night.

WARM UP AND COOL DOWN

Before beginning each workout, spend up to 5 minutes getting your heart rate up and blood flowing through your muscles. You can do this by jogging or marching in place, or by walking briskly for a short distance.

After your body is warm, perform a few minutes of more dynamic movements, such as Jumping Jacks, Air Squats, and High Knees. Spend a few minutes performing a couple sets of a handful of repetitions of each.

When starting your lifts, begin with 10 repetitions of an

unloaded bar. From there, gradually increase your weight in preparation of the work to come. We suggest 5 repetitions at a light weight, 5 repetitions at a slightly heavier weight, and then 5 repetitions at a moderate weight. This should provide a sufficient warm-up, yet not deplete you of needed energy.

When you complete each workout, spend a few minutes slowing your heart rate gradually by marching in place again or walking around the block, and then stretching.

THE FINE PRINT

The Farmer Gym Way and Farmer Gym do not provide medical advice. As with any exercise program, you should consult your physician before using it, especially if any of the following risk statuses apply to you: any pre-existing conditions that include but are not limited to a heart condition, pain in your chest from physical activity, dizziness or loss of consciousness when working out, known bone or joint problems, or taking prescription drugs. Farmer Gym workouts are intended for adults age 18 and over.

In addition, see your physician if you are a female over age 55, are a male over age 45, have a family history of heart disorder, have been a cigarette smoker in the past half-year, have led a sedentary life, are considered obese, are hypertensive, have high levels of lipids in your blood, or have a form of diabetes or other metabolic disorder. Likewise, when you are performing The Farmer Gym Way workouts, if you experience unusual pain, or if something doesn't feel right to you...STOP. Getting fit does not require injuries!

Farmer Gym has structured the workouts in this book to limit excessive back-to-back, repetitive muscle strain; however, there remains an extremely remote chance of excess muscle damage from overuse. If you begin feeling pain in your joints or experience unusual soreness or health issues, temporarily discontinue your exercise regimen and see a medical expert.

Results are not guaranteed. How much progress you see toward your fitness goals will depend on how often you exercise, how hard you push yourself while exercising, what your diet consists of, how active you are apart from working out, your genetic composition, and other factors. Working out with the Manual is an excellent start, but is not the only determinant of your health, fitness, and strength outcome.

Be smart. Stay hydrated by drinking water before, during, and after your workouts. Work out in a place that is a safe temperature. And if you begin feeling dizzy or light-headed, stop.

One more thing. It's important to conduct your workouts in places that allow for stable footing. If you are doing portions of your program workouts outside of a gym, make sure your exercise location accommodates safety, by choosing a flat, even surface that is not slippery or rocky.

Enough with the disclaimers. Let's start growing strong bodies!

THE EXERCISES

This section of The Farmer Gym Way contains detailed descriptions of how to perform each exercise included in the program's workouts, accompanied by photographs for illustration.

In most of the exercise descriptions below, you will see instructions to keep your spine straight and your core tight while performing the exercise. Your "core" consists of your abdominal muscles and your mid- to lower torso, which you should tighten by engaging the muscles. Similarly, keeping your spine straight requires awareness of aligning your vertebrae (or backbones) from your neck all the way down to your tailbone, without rounding your back or arching it and while keeping your chest up. We may also refer to this as a "neutral" spine. Keeping your spine straight and core tight is very important for protecting against injury, so we flag it up front here and repeat it throughout the exercise descriptions.

BENCH PRESS

* Lie with your head, back, and gluteus on the bench, and firmly plant your feet on the floor
* Place your hands on the bar wider than shoulder width
* Unrack the bar, and extend your arms to hold the bar over your chest
* In a controlled manner, descend the bar by bending your elbows until the bar reaches your chest
* Your elbows should be at a 45-degree angle from your ribcage, not flared outward in a T-like position
* From the bottom position, press upward until the bar is over your chest, then re-rack the bar

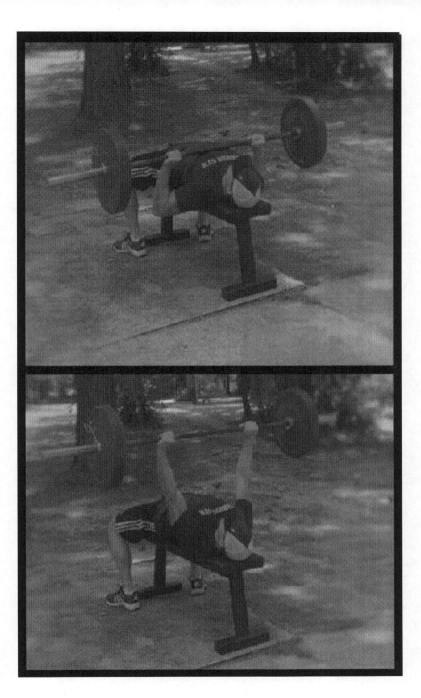

BOX JUMP

* Stand with your feet hip-width apart
* Keep your chest up and core tight
* Reach your arms down as you bend at your hips and knees
* After you descend to approximately the half-squat position, extend your arms up and jump into the air and toward the box
* While in the air, tuck your knees upward
* Land on the box with your knees bent
* Drive through your heels and gluteus to stand upright on the box, then step off and return to the starting position

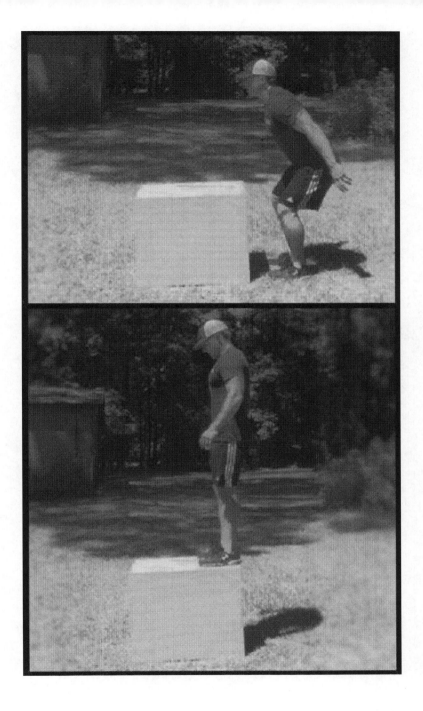

BURPEE

* Stand with your feet slightly wider than shoulder width
* Keep your chest up and core tight
* With your weight on your heels, squat down and place your hands on the ground
* With your weight on your hands and in your shoulders, jump and extend your body until you are in a Plank position
* Descend in a Push-up motion by bending your arms until your chest touches the ground
* Ascend to the Plank position by straightening your arms, and jump your knees forward to your chest
* Squat up, jump up into the air, and land in the starting position
(Scaled: Perform the Push-up portion from your knees)

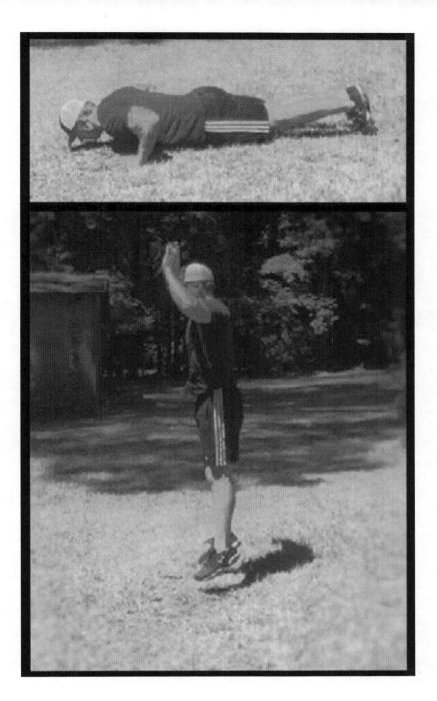

DEADLIFT

* Stand with your feet hip-width apart and your toes pointed slightly outward
* Place the bar over your feet and close to your shins
* In a controlled manner, set your body up by slightly bending your knees and shifting your hips back and down
* Your shoulders should be slightly ahead of the bar, and your lats should be tight before executing the movement
* After gripping the bar, lift your chest, and keep your chest up and head aligned with a neutral spine
* While maintaining a tight core and stable spine, ascend by straightening your knees while you push through your heels; once the bar passes your knees, begin to open your hips until you're standing up straight
* After standing upright, descend by reversing the ascension movement in a controlled manner

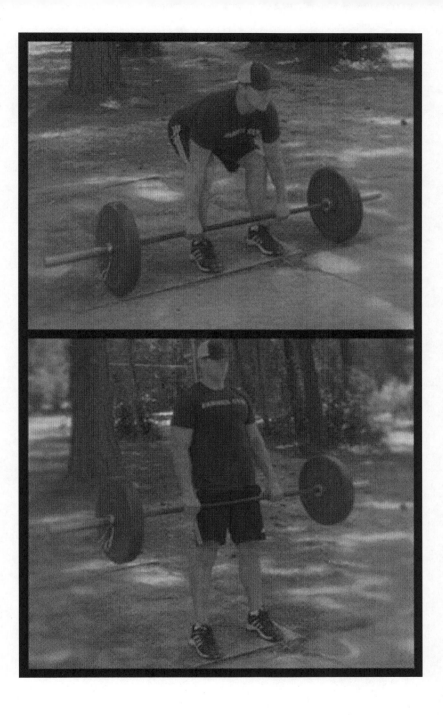

DEPTH PUSH-UP

* Lie face-down on the ground with your feet closer than hip-width apart
* Place the palms on the heads of the dumbbell, close to your shoulders
* With your toes on the ground and your elbows close to your side, push through your hands until your arms are extended
* Return to the ground slowly by bending your elbows until your chest reaches the ground

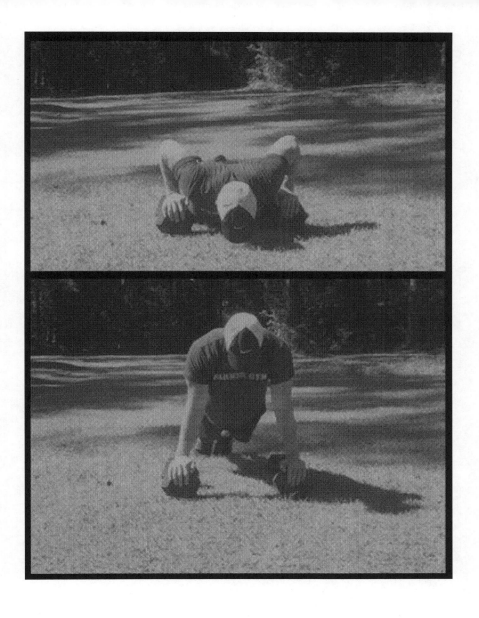

DIP

* Grab the bars and balance yourself with locked elbows
* Bend your arms and lower your body; your torso should begin to lean slightly forward
* Once your shoulders are at or below the level of your elbows, begin press upward and straighten your arms
* Expend your arms until you reach the starting position

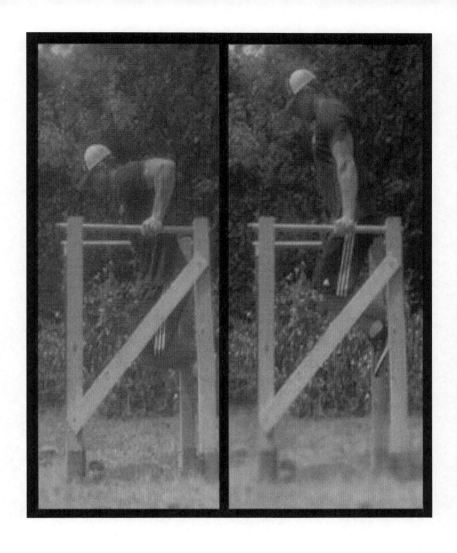

DUMBBELL BENCH PRESS

* Lie onto the bench with your head, back, and gluteus on the bench, and firmly plant your feet on the floor
* The dumbbells should be resting on your thighs
* From your thighs, raise each dumbbell to shoulder-level, one at a time (the dumbbells should be just to the sides of your chest)
* In a controlled manner, press the weights upward until they are over your chest and your arms are locked out
* Lower the weight in the same manner as you lifted it

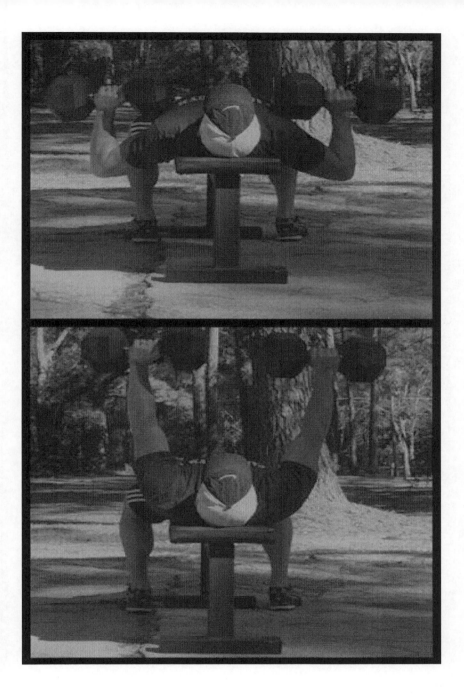

DUMBBELL DEADLIFT

* Stand with your feet hip-width apart and your toes pointed slightly outward
* Set your body up by slightly bending your knees and shifting your hips back and down
* Your shoulders should be slightly ahead of the dumbbells, and your lats should be tight before executing the movement
* Gripping the dumbbells, lift your chest, and keep your chest up and head aligned with a neutral spine
* While maintaining a tight core and stable spine, ascend by straightening your knees while you push through your heels
* Once the dumbbells pass above your knees, begin to open your hips until you're standing up straight
* After standing upright, descend by reversing the ascension movement in a controlled manner

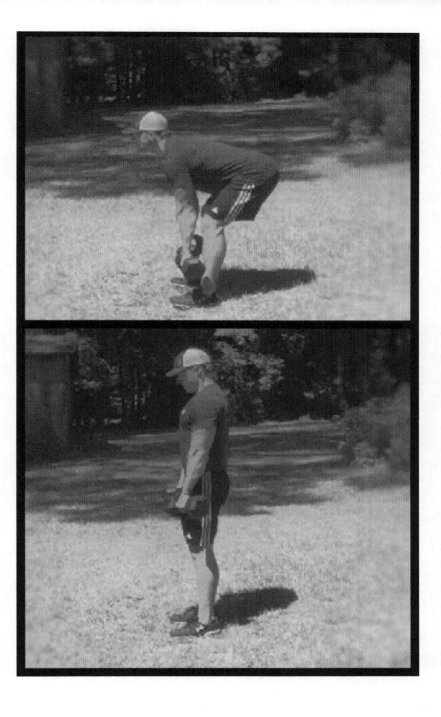

DUMBBELL LUNGE

* Stand upright with your feet together
* In a controlled manner, lift one leg off the ground and step forward
* Take a step, land with your heel first and toes pointing forward, and slowly shift the weight of your body onto your forward leg
* Maintain an upright torso, tight core, and straight spine
* Continue descending until your thigh is parallel to the ground, without letting your knee go past your toes
* Once in the lunge position, push off the front leg and return to the starting position, and alternate legs

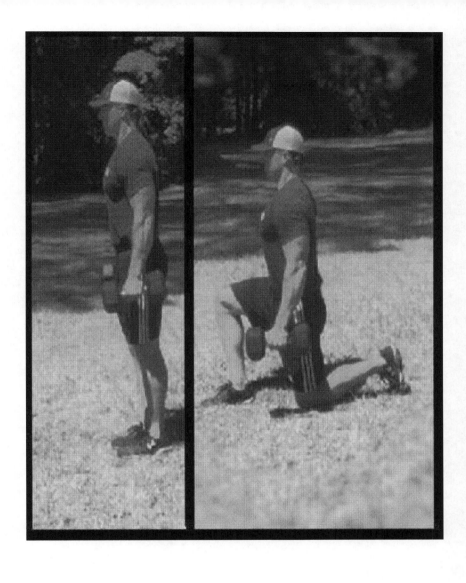

DUMBBELL OVERHEAD PRESS

* Stand with your feet hip-width apart
* Hold the dumbbells close to your body and just above your shoulders
* Hold your wrists straight and keep your elbows close to your body, with palms facing in
* With a tight core and straight back, drive the dumbbells up and over your head as you straighten your arms
* In a controlled manner, reverse the movement, and return the dumbbells to the starting position

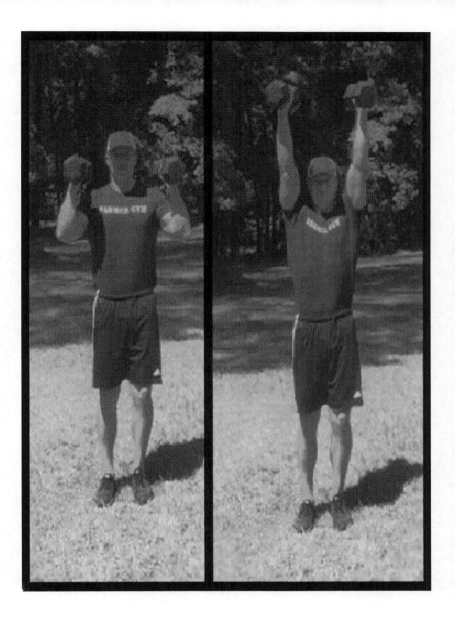

DUMBBELL SNATCH

* Stand with your feet shoulder-width apart and a dumbbell between your feet
* With your chest up and abs tight, grip the dumbbell by slightly bending your knees and shifting your hips back and down
* Press through the middle of your feet and drive the dumbbell upward
* Keep the dumbbell in a straight line, close to your body
* As the dumbbell moves upward, drive your elbow high until the dumbbell is overhead
* Catch the dumbbell at the top position with slightly bent knees, then stand upright
* In a controlled manner, reverse the movement and return the dumbbell to the ground

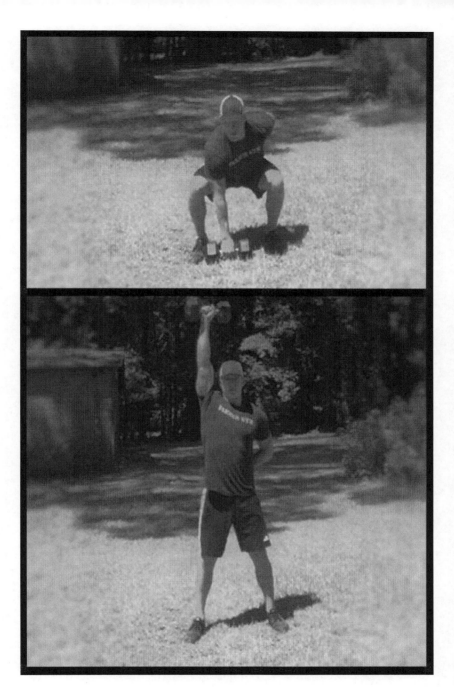

FARMER'S WALK

* Reach down to grab each dumbbell, and then stand up with them
* Make sure your back is tight while grasping the dumbbells
* With short, quick steps, walk with the dumbbells

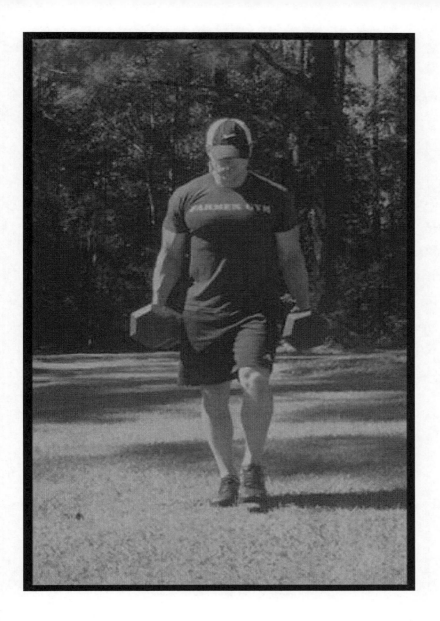

INVERTED ROW

* Position a bar around waist-height, and make sure it's firmly in place
* Place your hands on the bar at wider than shoulder width while hanging underneath it
* Your body should be straight, with core tight, heels on the ground, and arms fully extended
* Pull your chest up toward the bar by bending your arms while maintaining a rigid body
* Pause once your chest meets the bar, then reverse the movement to descend to the starting position

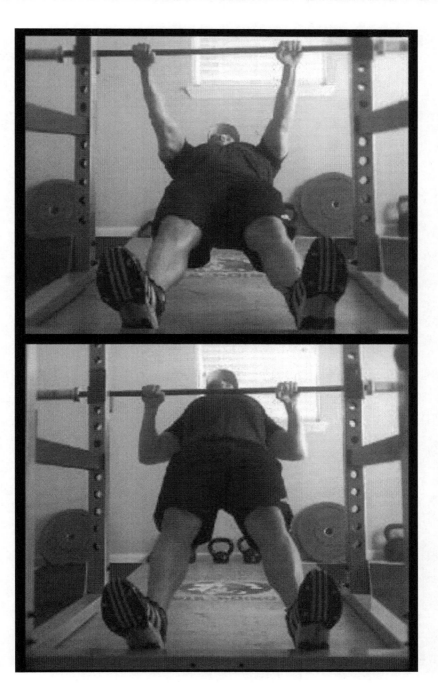

KETTLEBELL FRONT SQUAT

* Stand with your feet at shoulder width and toes pointed slightly outward
* Grab the Kettlebell by the handle with both hands, and hold it close to your chest with your elbows in
* Keep your chest and chin up, spine straight, and core tight
* Descend by pushing your hips and gluteus back and down
* Keep your weight on your heels
* Stop once your thighs are parallel to the ground, without letting your knees go past your toes or turn in
* Ascend by pushing through your heels
* Finish in the starting standing position

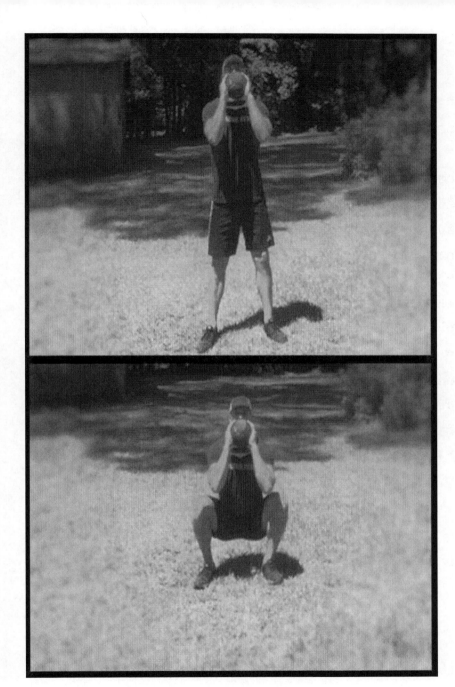

KETTLEBELL DEADLIFT HIGH-PULL

* Stand with your feet wider than shoulder width and toes pointed slightly outward
* Keep your chest and chin up, spine straight, and core tight
* Descend by pushing your hips and gluteus back and down, without letting your knees go past your toes or turn inward
* Keep your weight on your heels
* Grab the Kettlebell as you push through your heels and ascend to the top; at about midway, pull the Kettlebell up toward your chin by flaring your elbows out
* Keep your elbows held high once the Kettlebell reaches chin level
* Return the Kettlebell to the ground by reversing the ascension movement

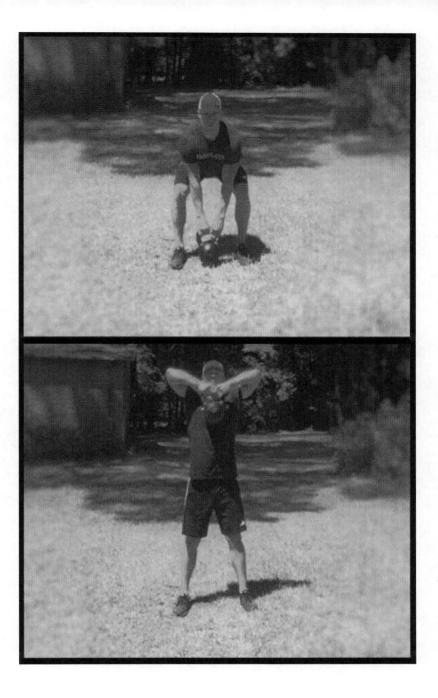

KETTLEBELL SQUAT PRESS

* Stand with your feet at shoulder width and toes pointed slightly outward
* Grab the Kettlebell by the handle with both hands, and hold it close to your chest with your elbows in
* Keep your chest and chin up, spine straight, and core tight
* Descend by pushing your hips and gluteus back and down
* Keep your weight on your heels
* Stop once your thighs are parallel to the ground, without letting your knees go past your toes or turn inward
* Ascend by pushing through your heels
* With your momentum, continue to drive the Kettlebell up and over your head, and lock your elbows out
* In a controlled motion, descend to the starting position

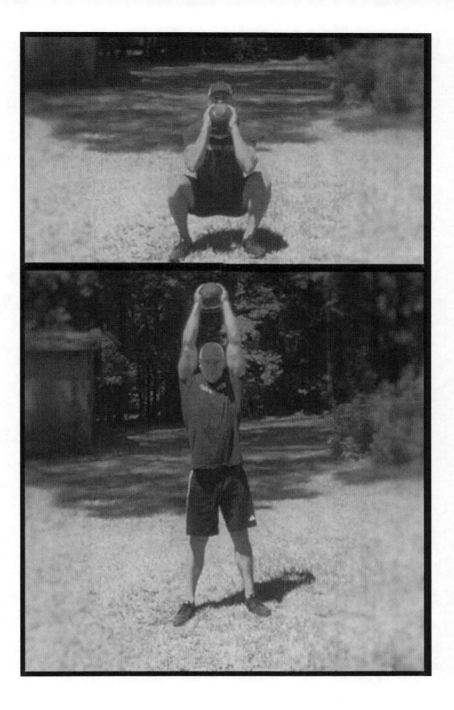

KETTLEBELL SWING

* Stand with your feet at shoulder width and toes pointed slightly outward, with the Kettlebell on the ground between your legs
* With your chest up and knees slightly bent, push your hips back and down
* Keep your weight on your heels
* Pull the Kettlebell close to your body and let it travel between the inside of your thighs
* Pop your hips and swing the Kettlebell forward
* Tighten your gluteus once your hips are open
* Let the Kettlebell use momentum and reach eye level
* Your arms should stay loose as the Kettlebell travels back to the starting position

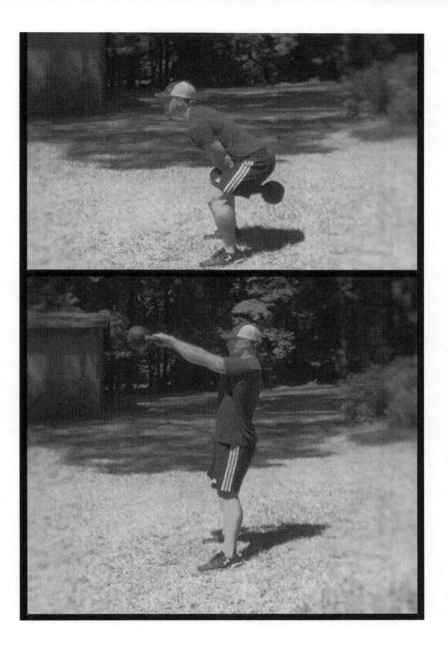

OVERHEAD PRESS

* Stand with your feet hip-width apart
* Place your hands on the bar just wider than shoulder width
* Hold your wrists straight and keep your elbows close to your body and pointed downward
* With a tight core and straight back, drive the bar up and over your head as you straighten your arms
* In a controlled manner, reverse the movement and return the bar to the starting position

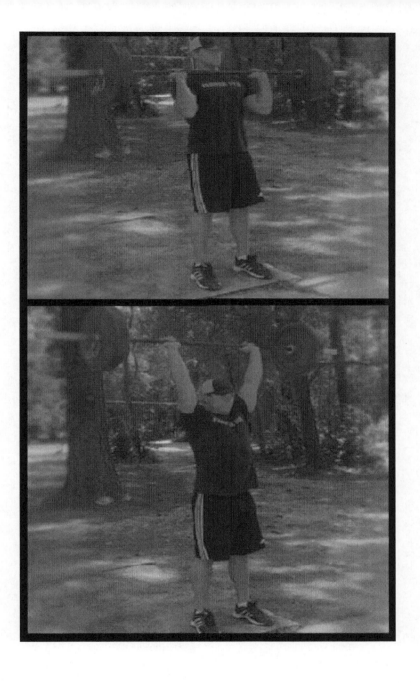

PULL-UP

(Scaled: Perform Lat Pull-downs or Inverted Row; for increased difficulty, perform Pull-ups with added weight)

* Hold the bar with your palms facing away from your body and hands wider than shoulder width
* Keep your core tight, spine straight, and shoulders engaged
* Your head should be in line with your spine
* With both arms extended above you, pull your body up in a controlled manner until your head is near bar level
* Upon reaching the top, slowly descend to the starting position
(Scaled: Perform Lat Pull-downs)

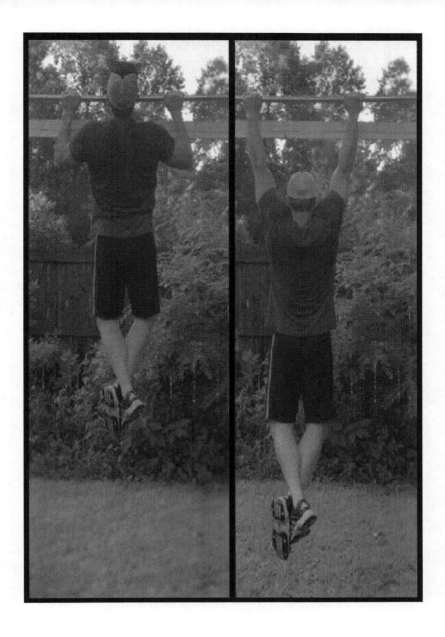

PUSH-UP

(Scaled: Perform from your knees)

* Lie face-down on the ground with your feet closer than hip-width apart
* Place the palms of your hands flat on the ground, close to your shoulders
* With your toes on the ground and your elbows close to your side, push through your hands until your arms are extended
* Return to the ground slowly by bending your elbows until your chest reaches the ground

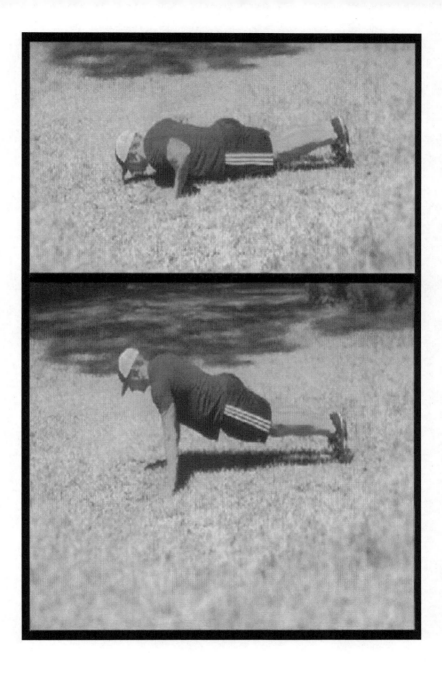

(BARBELL) ROW

* Stand over the bar with a hip-width stance, your knees slightly bent, and your mid-foot directly under the bar
* With your chest up, back straight, core tight, and hips elevated, reach down and grab the bar with a slightly wider than shoulder-width grasp
* Contract your back, then drive your elbows back so that the bar reaches your lower chest
* In a controlled manner, descend the bar by extending your elbows and returning the bar to the start position

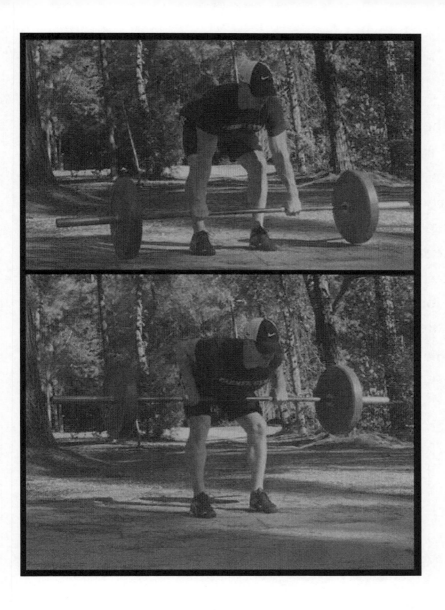

ROWER

* Hold the handle with extended arms, bent knees, and an upright chest
* Push through your feet, and once the handle passes your knees, pull backwards with your arms while leaning your torso slightly back
* Your elbows should drive back, and the handle should stop just below chest level
* The chain should remain straight throughout the pull
* Reverse the movement and return to the starting position by first extending your arms and leaning your torso forward, then bending your legs

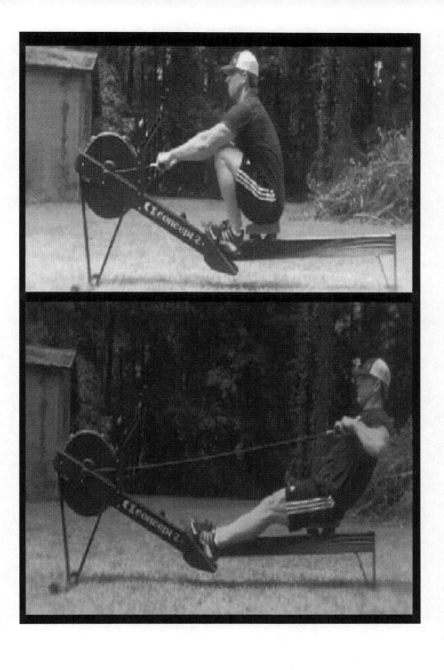

SIT-UP
(Scaled: Perform the Crunch)

* Lie down on your back with your knees bent and feet on the ground at hip width or slightly narrower
* With your elbows out wide, place your fingertips behind your head and squeeze your shoulder blades together
* With your gluteus and feet remaining on the ground, engage your stomach and raise your torso off the ground in a controlled manner until your torso has reached your thighs
* Descend by reversing the motion
* Keep your chin up and back straight throughout the exercise

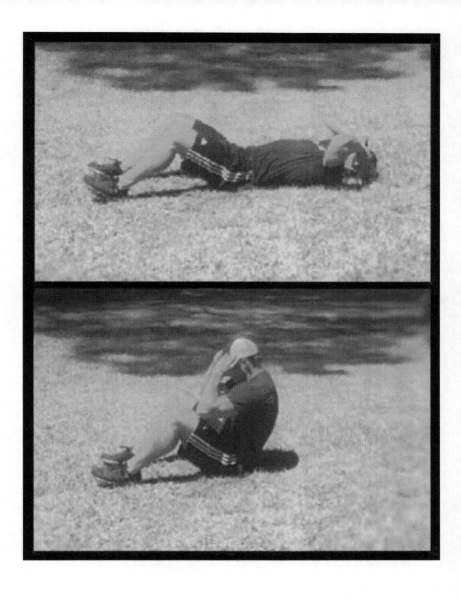

SQUAT

* Stand with your feet shoulder-width apart and toes pointed slightly outward
* Hold the bar with your hands wider than shoulder width and your elbows pointed down and slightly back
* Keep your chest up, spine straight, and core tight
* Descend by pushing your hips and gluteus back and down
* Keep your weight on your heels
* Stop once your thighs are at or below parallel to the ground
* Ascend by pushing through your heels
* Finish the squat in the starting position, standing up straight

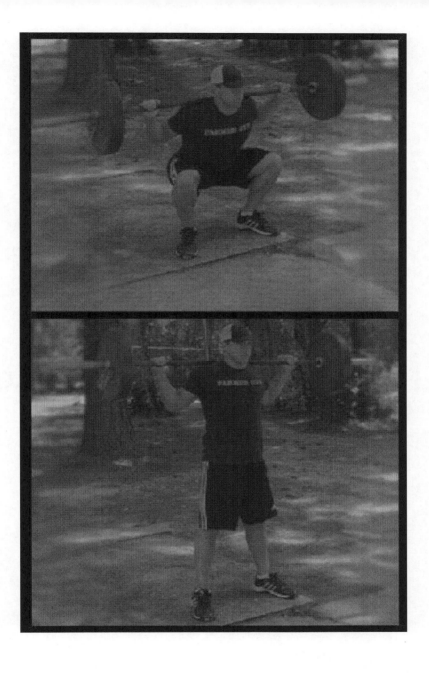

TUCK JUMP
(Scaled version of the Box Jump)

* Stand with your feet at hip width and toes pointed forward
* Keep your chest up and core tight
* Reach your arms down as you bend at your hips
* After you descend to approximately the half-squat position, swing your arms up and jump straight into the air
* While in the air, tuck your knees into your chest
* Land on the balls of your feet, with your knees bent, weight somewhat forward, and chest up
* Immediately spring back into the air and repeat the motion

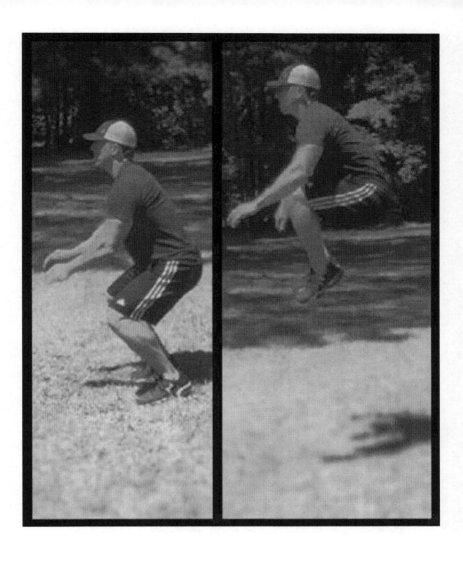

THE WORKOUTS

Week 1, Day 1 – Testing

Maximum Deadlift
*For those who have not performed a 1-repetition max in the past 2 months, execute a 5-repetition max and multiply the weight lifted by 87%.

Date	___/___/___	___/___/___
Weight Lifted		

Notes:

(Rest as needed)

2-minute Pull-ups
*For those unable to perform Pull-ups, execute Inverted Rows.

Date	___/___/___	___/___/___
Repetitions Completed		

Notes:

(Rest as needed)
*Continued on next page

Bodyweight Deadlifts
*Perform as many repetitions as possible; however, stop once form begins to fail, or when you are one or two reps shy of your true limit.

Date	___/___/___	___/___/___
Barbell Weight		
Repetitions Completed		

Notes:

(Rest as needed)

500-meter Row

Date	___/___/___	___/___/___
Time Completed		

Notes:

Week 1, Day 2 – Testing

Maximum Bench Press

*For those who have not performed a 1-repetition max in some time, execute a 5-repetition max and multiply the weight lifted by 87%.

Date	___/___/___	___/___/___
Weight Lifted		

Notes:

(Rest as needed)

800-meter Run

Date	___/___/___	___/___/___
Time Completed		

Notes:

(Rest as needed)
*Continued on next page

2-minute Push-ups

Date	___ / ___ / ___	___ / ___ / ___
Repetitions Completed		

Notes:

(Rest as needed)

7-minute Double-unders
*For those who are unable to perform Double-unders, execute Single-unders; for those who are unable to perform Single-unders, execute Jumping Jacks.

Date	___ / ___ / ___	___ / ___ / ___
Repetitions Completed		

Notes:

Week 1, Day 3 – Rest

Week 1, Day 4 – Testing

Maximum Squat
*For those who have not performed a 1-repetition max in some time, execute a 5-repetition max and multiply the weight lifted by 87%.

Date	___/___/___	___/___/___
Weight Lifted		

Notes:

(Rest as needed)

2-minute Sit-ups

Date	___/___/___	___/___/___
Repetitions Completed		

Notes:

(Rest as needed)
*Continued on next page

Bodyweight Squats
*Perform as many repetitions as possible; however, stop once form begins to fail, or when you are one or two reps shy of your true limit.

Date	___/___/___	___/___/___
Barbell Weight		
Repetitions Completed		

Notes:

(Rest as needed)

2,000-meter Row

Date	___/___/___	___/___/___
Time Completed		

Notes:

Week 1, Day 5 – Testing

Maximum Overhead Press
*For those who have not performed a 1-repetition max in some time, execute a 5-repetition max and multiply the weight lifted by 87%.

Date	___/___/___	___/___/___
Weight Lifted		

Notes:

(Rest as needed)

30-second Row

Date	___/___/___	___/___/___
Distance Completed		

Notes:

(Rest as needed)
*Continued on next page

7-minute Burpees

Date	____/____/____	____/____/____
Kettlebell Weight		
Repetitions Completed		

Notes:

(Rest as needed)

2-mile Run

Date	____/____/____	____/____/____
Time Completed		

Notes:

Week 1, Day 6 – Rest

Week 1, Day 7 – Rest

Week 2, Day 1 – Strength

Deadlift, 3 sets x 8 repetitions @ 70-75% 1RM

Date	___ / ___ / ___	___ / ___ / ___
Weight, Set 1		
Weight, Set 2		
Weight, Set 3		
Total Volume		

Strength notes:

Week 2, Day 1 – Conditioning

Perform as many Pull-ups as possible in 8 minutes. Every time you come off the bar, there is a 12 Kettlebell Front Squat penalty.
*For those unable to perform Pull-ups, execute Inverted Rows.

Male Kettlebell weight: 35-70#/Other#
Female Kettlebell weight: 15-45#/Other#

Date	__/__/__	__/__/__
Pull-ups Completed		
Kettlebell Weight		

(5-minute Rest)

Perform as many rounds as possible in 12 minutes:
500-meter Row
15 Burpees

Date	__/__/__	__/__/__
Meters Rowed		

Conditioning notes:

Week 2, Day 2 – Strength

Bench Press, 3 sets x 8 repetitions @ 70-75% 1RM

Date	___ / ___ / ___	___ / ___ / ___
Weight, Set 1		
Weight, Set 2		
Weight, Set 3		
Total Volume		

Strength notes:

Week 2, Day 2 – Conditioning

Perform 4 rounds:
25 Overhead Dumbbell Presses
50 Double-unders
800-meter Run
*45-minute time cap.
**For those unable to perform Double-unders, execute Single-unders; for those unable to perform Single-unders, execute Jumping Jacks.

Male Dumbbell weight: 25-50#/Other# (each Dumbbell)
Female Dumbbell weight: 15-30#/Other# (each Dumbbell)

Date	___/___/___	___/___/___
Time Completed		
Dumbbell Weight		

Conditioning notes:

Week 2, Day 3 – Rest

Week 2, Day 4 – Strength

Squat, 3 sets x 8 repetitions @ 70-75% 1RM

Date	___/___/___	___/___/___
Weight, Set 1		
Weight, Set 2		
Weight, Set 3		
Total Volume		

Strength notes:

Week 2, Day 4 – Conditioning

15 Deadlifts

30 Sit-ups

10 Deadlifts

20 Sit-ups

5 Deadlifts

10 Sit-ups

1-mile Run

30 Kettlebell Swings

60 Sit-ups

20 Kettlebell Swings

40 Sit-ups

10 Kettlebell Swings

20 Sit-ups

1-mile Run

*45-minute time cap.

Male and Female Barbell weight: 75% Bodyweight-
Bodyweight/Other#

Male Kettlebell weight: 35-70#/Other#

Female Kettlebell weight: 15-45#/Other#

Date	___ / ___ / ___	___ / ___ / ___
Time Completed		
Barbell Weight		
Kettlebell Weight		

Conditioning notes:

Week 2, Day 5 – Strength

Overhead Press, 3 sets x 8 repetitions @ 70-75% 1RM

Date	/ /	/ /
Weight, Set 1		
Weight, Set 2		
Weight, Set 3		
Total Volume		

Strength notes:

Week 2, Day 5 – Conditioning

In the following sequence, perform as many Dumbbell Bench Presses as possible, and Row as many meters as possible in 5 rounds:
As many Dumbbell Bench Presses as possible
(30-second Rest)
30-second Row
(2-minute Rest)

Male Dumbbell weight: 45-90#/Other# (each dumbbell)
Female Dumbbell weight: 15-45#/Other# (each dumbbell)

Date	___/___/___	___/___/___
DB BP, Round 1		
Meters Rowed, Round 1		
DB BP, Round 2		
Meters Rowed, Round 2		
DB BP, Round 3		
Meters Rowed, Round 3		
DB BP, Round 4		
Meters Rowed, Round 4		
DB BP, Round 5		
Meters Rowed, Round 5		
Total Push-ups		
Total Meters		
Dumbbell Weight		

Conditioning notes:

Week 2, Day 6 – Run

20-Minute Run for distance

Date	___/___/___	___/___/___
Distance		

Week 2, Day 7 – Rest

Week 3, Day 1 – Strength

Deadlift, 4 sets x 8 repetitions @ 75-80% 1RM
*Work up in weight so that the final set is challenging.

Date	__/__/__	__/__/__
Weight, Set 1		
Weight, Set 2		
Weight, Set 3		
Weight, Set 4		
Total Volume		

Strength notes:

Week 3, Day 1 – Conditioning

Perform 5 sets of as many repetitions of Pull-ups as possible. Rest 1 minute in between each set.

*For those unable to perform Pull-ups, execute Inverted Rows.

Date	___/___/___	___/___/___
Reps, Set 1		
Reps, Set 2		
Reps, Set 3		
Reps, Set 4		
Reps, Set 5		
Total Reps		

(5-minute Rest)

50 Kettlebell Squat Presses
800-meter Run
50 Kettlebell Squat Presses
*45-minute time cap.

Male Kettlebell weight: 35-70#/Other#
Female Kettlebell weight: 15-45#/Other#

Date	___/___/___	___/___/___
Time Completed		
Kettlebell Weight		

Conditioning notes:

Week 3, Day 2 – Strength

Bench Press, 4 sets x 8 repetitions @ 75-80% 1RM
*Work up in weight so that the final set is challenging.

Date	___/___/___	___/___/___
Weight, Set 1		
Weight, Set 2		
Weight, Set 3		
Weight, Set 4		
Total Volume		

Strength notes:

Week 3, Day 2 – Conditioning

Perform 5 sets of as many repetitions as possible of Dips. Rest 1 minute in between each set.

*For those unable to perform Dips, execute Push-ups

Date	___/___/___	___/___/___
Reps, Set 1		
Reps, Set 2		
Reps, Set 3		
Reps, Set 4		
Reps, Set 5		
Total Reps		

(5-minute Rest)

Perform 4 rounds:

Set your clock for 5 minutes, then perform 50 Double-unders; after your Double-unders, Row for as many meters as possible with the remainder of the 5 minutes. 2-minute rest in between each set.

*For those unable to perform Double-unders, execute Single-unders; for those unable to perform Single-unders, execute Jumping Jacks.

Date	___/___/___	___/___/___
Meters Rowed		

Conditioning notes:

Week 3, Day 3 – Rest

Week 3, Day 4 – Strength

Squat, 4 sets x 8 repetitions @ 75-80% 1RM
*Work up in weight so that the final set is challenging.

Date	___/___/___	___/___/___
Weight, Set 1		
Weight, Set 2		
Weight, Set 3		
Weight, Set 4		
Total Volume		

Strength notes:

Week 3, Day 4 – Conditioning

Perform as many repetitions of the following as possible in 5 rounds:
1-minute Dumbbell Snatches
1-minute Sit-ups
(30-second Rest)

Male Dumbbell weight: 35-70#/Other#
Female Dumbbell weight: 20-45#/Other#

Date	___/___/___	___/___/___
Repetitions Completed		
Dumbbell Weight		

(5-minute rest)

Perform 2 rounds of the following for time:
25 Kettlebell Deadlift High-pulls
800-meter Run
800-meter Row
*45-minute time cap.

Male Kettlebell weight: 35-70#/Other#
Female Kettlebell weight: 20-45#/Other#

Date	___/___/___	___/___/___
Time Completed		
Kettlebell Weight		

Conditioning notes:

Week 3, Day 5 – Strength

Overhead Press, 4 sets x 8 repetitions @ 75-80% 1RM
*Work up in weight so that the final set is challenging.

Date	__/__/__	__/__/__
Weight, Set 1		
Weight, Set 2		
Weight, Set 3		
Weight, Set 4		
Total Volume		

Strength notes:

Week 3, Day 5 – Conditioning

Perform as many rounds as possible in 30 minutes:

50 Push-ups

10 Box Jumps

10 Burpees

400-meter Run

Male Box height: 20-24"/Tuck Jump

Female Box height: 20"/Tuck Jump

Date	___/___/___	___/___/___
Rounds Completed		
Box Jump Height		

Conditioning notes:

Week 3, Day 6 – Run

25-minute Run for distance

Date	___ / ___ / ___	___ / ___ / ___
Distance		

Week 3, Day 7 – Rest

Week 4, Day 1 – Strength

Deadlift, 4 sets x 8 repetitions @ 75-80% 1RM
*Work up in weight so that the final two sets are challenging.

Date	___/___/___	___/___/___
Weight, Set 1		
Weight, Set 2		
Weight, Set 3		
Weight, Set 4		
Total Volume		

Strength notes:

Week 4, Day 1 – Conditioning

10-minute, 5-repetition EMOM (every minute on the minute) Squat. At minute 0, execute 5 reps of the Squat; upon completion, rest the remainder of the minute. At minute 1, once again Squat 5 reps; upon completion, rest the remainder of the minute. Continue this process until you have completed 10 rounds. If you get to a point where you can no longer perform 5 repetitions, stop.

Male and Female Squat weight: 65% Bodyweight-Bodyweight/Other#

Date	___/___/___	___/___/___
Repetitions Completed		
Barbell Weight		

(5-minute Rest)

Perform 3 rounds:
25 Kettlebell Swings
25 Pull-ups
400-meter Run
*For those unable to perform Pull-ups, execute Inverted Rows.

Male Kettlebell weight: 45-70#/Other#
Female Kettlebell weight: 20-45#/Other#

Date	___/___/___	___/___/___
Time Completed		
Kettlebell Weight		

Conditioning note:

Week 4, Day 2 – Strength

Bench Press, 4 sets x 8 repetitions @ 75-80% 1RM
*Work up in weight so that the final two sets are challenging.

Date	___/___/___	___/___/___
Weight, Set 1		
Weight, Set 2		
Weight, Set 3		
Weight, Set 4		
Total Volume		

Strength notes:

Week 4, Day 2 – Conditioning

8 Overhead Presses
8 Box Jumps
30 Sit-ups
300-meter Row
8 Overhead Presses (Add 5 pounds)
8 Box Jumps
30 Sit-ups
300-meter Row
8 Overhead Presses (Add 5 pounds)
8 Box Jumps
30 Sit-ups
300-meter Row
...and so on and so forth, until you can no longer perform 8
Overhead Presses or until you have worked out for 30 minutes.

Male Barbell starting weight begins at 50-60% of Max Press/Other#
Female Barbell starting weight begins at 30-40% of Max
Press/Other#
Male Box height: 20-24"/Tuck Jump
Female Box height: 20"/Tuck Jump

Date	__/__/__	__/__/__
Rounds Completed		
Starting Barbell Weight		
Box Jump Height		

Conditioning notes:

Week 4, Day 3 – Rest

Week 4, Day 4 – Strength

Squat, 4 sets x 8 repetitions @ 75-80% 1RM
*Work up in weight so that the final two sets are challenging.

Date	___ / ___ / ___	___ / ___ / ___
Weight, Set 1		
Weight, Set 2		
Weight, Set 3		
Weight, Set 4		
Total Volume		

Strength notes:

Week 4, Day 4 – Conditioning

Perform 3 rounds of the following:

15 Deadlifts

15 Burpees

Male Barbell weight: 185-225#/Other#

Female Barbell weight: 95-135#/Other#

Date	___/___/___	___/___/___
Time Completed		
Deadlift Weight		

(5-minute Rest)

2,000-meter Row

Time Completed		

Conditioning notes:

Week 4, Day 5 – Strength:

Overhead Press, 4 sets x 8 repetitions @ 75-80% 1RM
*Work up in weight so that the final two sets are challenging.

Date	___ / ___ / ___	___ / ___ / ___
Weight, Set 1		
Weight, Set 2		
Weight, Set 3		
Weight, Set 4		
Total Volume		

Strength notes:

Week 4, Day 5 – Conditioning

Perform 2 rounds of the following:
10 Dumbbell Bench Presses
10 Barbell Rows
9 Dumbbell Bench Presses
9 Barbell Rows
...and so on and so forth, until the round of 1 repetitions is complete.

Male Dumbbell weight: 45-90#/Other# (each dumbbell)
Female Dumbbell weight: 15-45#/Other# (each dumbbell)
Male Barbell weight: 40-60% Bodyweight/Other#
Female Barbell weight: 20-40% Bodyweight/Other#

Date	__/__/__	__/__/__
Time Performed		
Dumbbell Weight		
Barbell Weight		

(5-minute Rest)

Perform 8 minutes of the Farmer's Walk for distance. Every time you place the weight down, there is a 10 Depth Push-up penalty.

Male Dumbbell weight: 45-70#/Other# (each dumbbell)
Female Dumbbell weight: 20-45#/Other# (each dumbbell)

Distance Completed		

Conditioning Notes:

Week 4, Day 6 – Run

30-minute Run for distance

Date	___ / ___ / ___	___ / ___ / ___
Distance		

Week 4, Day 7 – Rest

Week 5, Day 1 – Conditioning (No Strength)

Perform for 30 minutes:
10 Dumbbell Lunges (5 per leg)
5 Dumbbell Deadlifts (same weight)
20 Sit-ups

Male Dumbbell weight: 35-70#/Other# (each dumbbell)
Female Dumbbell weight: 15-45#/Other# (each dumbbell)

Date	___/___/___	___/___/___
Rounds Completed		
Dumbbell Weight		

Conditioning notes:

Week 5, Day 2 – Conditioning (No Strength)

Perform for 30 minutes:
5 Pull-ups
15 Push-ups
25 Double-unders
*For those unable to perform Pull-ups, execute Inverted Rows.
**For those who are unable to perform Double-unders, execute
Single-unders; for those who are unable to perform Single-unders,
execute Jumping Jacks.

Date	___/___/___	___/___/___
Rounds Completed		

Conditioning notes:

Week 5, Day 3 – Rest

Week 5, Day 4 – Run

20-minute Run for distance

Date	___ / ___ / ___	___ / ___ / ___
Distance		

Week 5, Day 5 – Row

20-minute Row for distance

Date	___ / ___ / ___	___ / ___ / ___
Distance		

Week 5, Day 6 – Rest

Week 5, Day 7 – Rest

Week 6, Day 1 – Strength

Deadlift, 4 sets x 5 repetitions @ 80-85% 1RM

Date	___/___/___	___/___/___
Weight, Set 1		
Weight, Set 2		
Weight, Set 3		
Weight, Set 4		
Total Volume		

Strength notes:

Week 6, Day 1 – Conditioning

Perform as many Pull-ups as possible in 8 minutes. Every time you come off the bar, there is a 12 Kettlebell Front Squat penalty.
*For those unable to perform Pull-ups, execute Inverted Rows.

Male Kettlebell weight: 35-70#/Other#
Female Kettlebell weight: 15-45#/Other#

Date	__ / __ / __	__ / __ / __
Pull-ups Completed		
Kettlebell Weight		

(5-minute Rest)

Perform as many rounds as possible in 12 minutes:
500-meter Row
15 Burpees

Date	__ / __ / __	__ / __ / __
Meters Rowed		

Conditioning notes:

Week 6, Day 2 – Strength

Bench Press, 4 sets x 5 repetitions @ 80-85% 1RM

Date	__/__/__	__/__/__
Weight, Set 1		
Weight, Set 2		
Weight, Set 3		
Weight, Set 4		
Total Volume		

Strength notes:

Week 6, Day 2 – Conditioning

Perform 4 rounds:
25 Overhead Dumbbell Presses
50 Double-unders
800-meter Run
*45-minute time cap.
**For those unable to perform Double-unders, execute Single-unders; for those unable to perform Single-unders, execute Jumping Jacks.

Male Dumbbell weight: 25-50#/Other# (each Dumbbell)
Female Dumbbell weight: 15-30#/Other# (each Dumbbell)

Date	___ / ___ / ___	___ / ___ / ___
Time Completed		
Dumbbell Weight		

Conditioning notes:

Week 6, Day 3 – Rest

Week 6, Day 4 – Strength

Squat, 4 sets x 5 repetitions @ 80-85% 1RM

Date	___/___/___	___/___/___
Weight, Set 1		
Weight, Set 2		
Weight, Set 3		
Weight, Set 4		
Total Volume		

Strength notes:

Week 6, Day 4 – Conditioning

15 Deadlifts
30 Sit-ups
10 Deadlifts
20 Sit-ups
5 Deadlifts
10 Sit-ups
1-mile Run
30 Kettlebell Swings
60 Sit-ups
20 Kettlebell Swings
40 Sit-ups
10 Kettlebell Swings
20 Sit-ups
1-mile Run
*45-minute time cap.

Male and Female Barbell weight: 75% Bodyweight-
Bodyweight/Other#
Male Kettlebell weight: 35-70#/Other#
Female Kettlebell weight: 15-45#/Other#

Date	___ / ___ / ___	___ / ___ / ___
Time Completed		
Barbell Weight		
Kettlebell Weight		

Conditioning notes:

Week 6, Day 5 – Strength

Overhead Press, 4 sets x 5 repetitions @ 80-85% 1RM

Date	__/__/__	__/__/__
Weight, Set 1		
Weight, Set 2		
Weight, Set 3		
Weight, Set 4		
Total Volume		

Strength notes:

Week 6, Day 5 – Conditioning

Perform as many Dumbbell Bench Presses as possible, and Row as many meters as possible in 5 rounds:

As many Dumbbell Bench Presses as possible

(30-second Rest)

30-second Row

(2-minute Rest)

Male Dumbbell weight: 45-90#/Other# (each dumbbell)

Female Dumbbell weight: 15-45#/Other# (each dumbbell)

Date	___/___/___	___/___/___
DB BP, Round 1		
Meters Rowed, Round 1		
DB BP, Round 2		
Meters Rowed, Round 2		
DB BP, Round 3		
Meters Rowed, Round 3		
DB BP, Round 4		
Meters Rowed, Round 4		
DB BP, Round 5		
Meters Rowed, Round 5		
Total Push-ups		
Total Meters		
Dumbbell Weight		

Conditioning notes:

Week 6, Day 6 – Run

20-Minute Run for distance

Date	___/___/___	___/___/___
Distance		

Week 6, Day 7 – Rest

Week 7, Day 1 – Strength

Deadlift, 5 sets x 5 repetitions @ 82-87% 1RM
*Work up in weight so that the final set is challenging.

Date	___ / ___ / ___	___ / ___ / ___
Weight, Set 1		
Weight, Set 2		
Weight, Set 3		
Weight, Set 4		
Weight, Set 5		
Total Volume		

Strength notes:

Week 7, Day 1 – Conditioning

Perform 5 sets of as many repetitions of Pull-ups as possible. Rest 1 minute in between each set.

*For those unable to perform Pull-ups, execute Inverted Rows.

Date	___/___/___	___/___/___
Reps, Set 1		
Reps, Set 2		
Reps, Set 3		
Reps, Set 4		
Reps, Set 5		
Total Reps		

(5-minute Rest)

50 Kettlebell Squat Presses
800-meter Run
50 Kettlebell Squat Presses
*45-minute time cap.

Male Kettlebell weight: 35-70#/Other#
Female Kettlebell weight: 15-45#/Other#

Date	___/___/___	___/___/___
Time Completed		
Kettlebell Weight		

Conditioning notes:

Week 7, Day 2 – Strength

Bench Press, 5 sets x 5 repetitions @ 82-87% 1RM
*Work up in weight so that the final set is challenging.

Date	___ / ___ / ___	___ / ___ / ___
Weight, Set 1		
Weight, Set 2		
Weight, Set 3		
Weight, Set 4		
Weight, Set 5		
Total Volume		

Strength notes:

Week 7, Day 2 – Conditioning

Perform 5 sets of as many repetitions as possible of Dips. Rest 1 minute in between each set.

*For those unable to perform Dips, execute Push-ups

Date	___/___/___	___/___/___
Reps, Set 1		
Reps, Set 2		
Reps, Set 3		
Reps, Set 4		
Reps, Set 5		
Total Reps		

(5-minute Rest)

Perform 4 rounds:

Set your clock for 5 minutes, then perform 50 Double-unders; after your Double-unders, Row for as many meters as possible with the remainder of the 5 minutes. 2-minute rest in between each set.

*For those unable to perform Double-unders, execute Single-unders; for those unable to perform Single-unders, execute Jumping Jacks.

Date	___/___/___	___/___/___
Meters Rowed		

Conditioning notes:

Week 7, Day 3 – Rest

Week 7, Day 4 – Strength

Squat, 5 sets x 5 repetitions @ 82-87% 1RM
*Work up in weight so that the final set is challenging.

Date	___ / ___ / ___	___ / ___ / ___
Weight, Set 1		
Weight, Set 2		
Weight, Set 3		
Weight, Set 4		
Weight, Set 5		
Total Volume		

Strength notes:

Week 7, Day 4 – Conditioning

Perform as many repetitions of the following as possible in 5 rounds:
1-minute Dumbbell Snatches
1-minute Sit-ups
(30-second Rest)

Male Dumbbell weight: 35-70#/Other#
Female Dumbbell weight: 20-45#/Other#

Date	___/___/___	___/___/___
Repetitions Completed		
Dumbbell Weight		

(5-minute rest)

Perform 2 rounds of the following for time:
25 Kettlebell Deadlift High-pulls
800-meter Run
800-meter Row
*45-minute time cap.

Male Kettlebell weight: 35-70#/Other#
Female Kettlebell weight: 20-45#/Other#

Date	___/___/___	___/___/___
Time Completed		
Kettlebell Weight		

Conditioning notes:

Week 7, Day 5 – Strength

Overhead Press, 5 sets x 5 repetitions @ 82-87% 1RM
*Work up in weight so that the final set is challenging.

Date	___ / ___ / ___	___ / ___ / ___
Weight, Set 1		
Weight, Set 2		
Weight, Set 3		
Weight, Set 4		
Weight, Set 5		
Total Volume		

Strength notes:

Week 7, Day 5 – Conditioning

Perform as many rounds as possible in 30 minutes:

50 Push-ups

10 Box Jumps

10 Burpees

400-meter Run

Male Box height: 20-24"/Tuck Jump

Female Box height: 20"/Tuck Jump

Date	___/___/___	___/___/___
Rounds Completed		
Box Jump Height		

Conditioning notes:

Week 7, Day 6 – Run

25-minute Run for distance

Date	___/___/___	___/___/___
Distance		

Week 7, Day 7 – Rest

Week 8, Day 1 – Strength

Deadlift, 5 sets x 5 repetitions @ 82-87% 1RM
*Work up in weight so that the final two sets are challenging.

Date	___/___/___	___/___/___
Weight, Set 1		
Weight, Set 2		
Weight, Set 3		
Weight, Set 4		
Weight, Set 5		
Total Volume		

Strength notes:

Week 8, Day 1 – Conditioning

10-minute, 5-repetition EMOM (every minute on the minute) Squat. At minute 0, execute 5 reps of the Squat; upon completion, rest the remainder of the minute. At minute 1, once again Squat 5 reps; upon completion, rest the remainder of the minute. Continue this process until you have completed 10 rounds. If you get to a point where you can no longer perform 5 repetitions, stop.

Male and Female Squat weight: 65% Bodyweight-Bodyweight/Other#

Date	__/__/__	__/__/__
Repetitions Completed		
Barbell Weight		

(5-minute Rest)

Perform 3 rounds:
25 Kettlebell Swings
25 Pull-ups
400-meter Run
*For those unable to perform Pull-ups, execute Inverted Rows.

Male Kettlebell weight: 35-70#/Other#
Female Kettlebell weight: 20-45#/Other#

Date	__/__/__	__/__/__
Time Completed		
Kettlebell Weight		

Conditioning note:

Week 8, Day 2 – Strength

Bench Press, 5 sets x 5 repetitions @ 82-87% 1RM
*Work up in weight so that the final two sets are challenging.

Date	___/___/___	___/___/___
Weight, Set 1		
Weight, Set 2		
Weight, Set 3		
Weight, Set 4		
Weight, Set 5		
Total Volume		

Strength notes:

Week 8, Day 2 – Conditioning

8 Overhead Presses

8 Box Jumps

30 Sit-ups

300-meter Row

8 Overhead Presses (Add 5 pounds)

8 Box Jumps

30 Sit-ups

300-meter Row

8 Overhead Presses (Add 5 pounds)

8 Box Jumps

30 Sit-ups

300-meter Row

...and so on and so forth, until you can no longer perform 8 Overhead Presses or until you have worked out for 30 minutes.

Male Barbell starting weight begins at 50-60% of Max Press/Other#

Female Barbell starting weight begins at 30-40% of Max Press/Other#

Male Box height: 20-24"/Tuck Jump

Female Box height: 20"/Tuck Jump

Date	___/___/___	___/___/___
Rounds Completed		
Starting Barbell Weight		
Box Jump Height		

Conditioning notes:

Week 8, Day 3 – Rest

Week 8, Day 4 – Strength

Squat, 5 sets x 5 repetitions @ 82-87% 1RM
*Work up in weight so that the final two sets are challenging.

Date	___/___/___	___/___/___
Weight, Set 1		
Weight, Set 2		
Weight, Set 3		
Weight, Set 4		
Weight, Set 5		
Total Volume		

Strength notes:

Week 8, Day 4 – Conditioning

Perform 3 rounds of the following:

15 Deadlifts

15 Burpees

Male Barbell weight: 185-225#/Other#

Female Barbell weight: 95-135#/Other#

Date	___/___/___	___/___/___
Time Completed		
Deadlift Weight		

(5-minute Rest)

2,000-meter Row

Time Completed		

Conditioning notes:

Week 8, Day 5 – Strength:

Overhead Press, 5 sets x 5 repetitions @ 82-87% 1RM
*Work up in weight so that the final two sets are challenging.

Date	___ / ___ / ___	___ / ___ / ___
Weight, Set 1		
Weight, Set 2		
Weight, Set 3		
Weight, Set 4		
Weight, Set 5		
Total Volume		

Strength notes:

Week 8, Day 5 – Conditioning

Perform 2 rounds of the following:
10 Dumbbell Bench Presses
10 Barbell Rows
9 Dumbbell Bench Presses
9 Barbell Rows
...and so on and so forth, until the round of 1 repetitions is complete.

Male Dumbbell weight: 45-90#/Other# (each dumbbell)
Female Dumbbell weight: 15-45#/Other# (each dumbbell)
Male Barbell weight: 40-60% Bodyweight/Other#
Female Barbell weight: 20-40% Bodyweight/Other#

Date	___/___/___	___/___/___
Time Performed		
Dumbbell Weight		
Barbell Weight		

(5-minute Rest)

Perform 8 minutes of the Farmer's Walk for distance. Every time you place the weight down, there is a 10 Depth Push-up penalty.

Male Dumbbell weight: 45-70#/Other# (each dumbbell)
Female Dumbbell weight: 20-45#/Other# (each dumbbell)

Distance Completed		

Conditioning Notes:

Week 8, Day 6 – Run

30-minute Run for distance

Date	___ / ___ / ___	___ / ___ / ___
Distance		

Week 8, Day 7 – Rest

Week 9, Day 1 – Conditioning (No Strength)

Perform for 30 minutes:
10 Dumbbell Lunges (5 per leg)
5 Dumbbell Deadlifts (same weight)
20 Sit-ups

Male Dumbbell weight: 35-70#/Other# (each dumbbell)
Female Dumbbell weight: 15-45#/Other# (each dumbbell)

Date	___/___/___	___/___/___
Rounds Completed		
Dumbbell Weight		

Conditioning notes:

Week 9, Day 2 – Conditioning (No Strength)

Perform for 30 minutes:
5 Pull-ups
15 Push-ups
25 Double-unders
*For those unable to perform Pull-ups, execute Inverted Rows.
**For those who are unable to perform Double-unders, execute Single-unders; for those who are unable to perform Single-unders, execute Jumping Jacks.

Date	___ / ___ / ___	___ / ___ / ___
Rounds Completed		

Conditioning notes:

<u>Week 9, Day 3 – Rest</u>

Week 9, Day 4 – Run

20-minute Run for distance

Date	____ / ____ / ____	____ / ____ / ____
Distance		

Week 9, Day 5 – Row

20-minute Row for distance

Date	_____ / _____ / _____	_____ / _____ / _____
Distance		

<u>**Week 9, Day 6 – Rest**</u>

Week 10, Day 1 – Strength

Deadlift, 5 sets x 3 repetitions @ 87-90% 1RM

Date	__/__/__	__/__/__
Weight, Set 1		
Weight, Set 2		
Weight, Set 3		
Weight, Set 4		
Weight, Set 5		
Total Volume		

Strength notes:

Week 10, Day 1 – Conditioning

Perform as many Pull-ups as possible in 8 minutes. Every time you come off the bar, there is a 12 Kettlebell Front Squat penalty.
*For those unable to perform Pull-ups, execute Inverted Rows.

Male Kettlebell weight: 35-70#/Other#
Female Kettlebell weight: 15-45#/Other#

Date	___/___/___	___/___/___
Pull-ups Completed		
Kettlebell Weight		

(5-minute Rest)

Perform as many rounds as possible in 12 minutes:
500-meter Row
15 Burpees

Date	___/___/___	___/___/___
Meters Rowed		

Conditioning notes:

Week 10, Day 2 – Strength

Bench Press, 5 sets x 3 repetitions @ 87-90% 1RM

Date	___/___/___	___/___/___
Weight, Set 1		
Weight, Set 2		
Weight, Set 3		
Weight, Set 4		
Weight, Set 5		
Total Volume		

Strength notes:

Week 10, Day 2 – Conditioning

Perform 4 rounds:
25 Overhead Dumbbell Presses
50 Double-unders
800-meter Run
*45-minute time cap.
**For those unable to perform Double-unders, execute Single-unders; for those unable to perform Single-unders, execute Jumping Jacks.

Male Dumbbell weight: 25-50#/Other# (each Dumbbell)
Female Dumbbell weight: 15-30#/Other# (each Dumbbell)

Date	___/___/___	___/___/___
Time Completed		
Dumbbell Weight		

Conditioning notes:

Week 10, Day 3 – Rest

Week 10, Day 4 – Strength

Squat, 5 sets x 3 repetitions @ 87-90% 1RM

Date	___ / ___ / ___	___ / ___ / ___
Weight, Set 1		
Weight, Set 2		
Weight, Set 3		
Weight, Set 4		
Weight, Set 5		
Total Volume		

Strength notes:

Week 10, Day 4 – Conditioning

15 Deadlifts

30 Sit-ups

10 Deadlifts

20 Sit-ups

5 Deadlifts

10 Sit-ups

1-mile Run

30 Kettlebell Swings

60 Sit-ups

20 Kettlebell Swings

40 Sit-ups

10 Kettlebell Swings

20 Sit-ups

1-mile Run

*45-minute time cap.

Male and Female Barbell weight: 75% Bodyweight-Bodyweight/Other#

Male Kettlebell weight: 35-70#/Other#

Female Kettlebell weight: 15-45#/Other#

Date	___ / ___ / ___	___ / ___ / ___
Time Completed		
Barbell Weight		
Kettlebell Weight		

Conditioning notes:

Week 10, Day 5 – Strength

Overhead Press, 5 sets x 3 repetitions @ 87-90% 1RM

Date	___ / ___ / ___	___ / ___ / ___
Weight, Set 1		
Weight, Set 2		
Weight, Set 3		
Weight, Set 4		
Weight, Set 5		
Total Volume		

Strength notes:

Week 10, Day 5 – Conditioning

Perform as many Dumbbell Bench Presses as possible, and Row as many meters as possible in 5 rounds:
As many Dumbbell Bench Presses as possible
(30-second Rest)
30-second Row
(2-minute Rest)

Male Dumbbell weight: 45-90#/Other# (each dumbbell)
Female Dumbbell weight: 15-45#/Other# (each dumbbell)

Date	___/___/___	___/___/___
DB BP, Round 1		
Meters Rowed, Round 1		
DB BP, Round 2		
Meters Rowed, Round 2		
DB BP, Round 3		
Meters Rowed, Round 3		
DB BP, Round 4		
Meters Rowed, Round 4		
DB BP, Round 5		
Meters Rowed, Round 5		
Total Push-ups		
Total Meters		
Dumbbell Weight		

Conditioning notes:

Week 10, Day 6 – Run

20-Minute Run for distance

Date	___/___/___	___/___/___
Distance		

Week 10, Day 7 – Rest

Week 11, Day 1 – Strength

Deadlift, 6 sets x 3 repetitions @ 90-92% 1RM
*Work up in weight so that the final set is challenging.

Date	___ / ___ / ___	___ / ___ / ___
Weight, Set 1		
Weight, Set 2		
Weight, Set 3		
Weight, Set 4		
Weight, Set 5		
Weight, Set 6		
Total Volume		

Strength notes:

Week 11, Day 1 – Conditioning

Perform 5 sets of as many repetitions of Pull-ups as possible. Rest 1 minute in between each set.

*For those unable to perform Pull-ups, execute Inverted Rows.

Date	__/__/__	__/__/__
Reps, Set 1		
Reps, Set 2		
Reps, Set 3		
Reps, Set 4		
Reps, Set 5		
Total Reps		

(5-minute Rest)

50 Kettlebell Squat Presses
800-meter Run
50 Kettlebell Squat Presses
*45-minute time cap.

Male Kettlebell weight: 35-70#/Other#
Female Kettlebell weight: 15-45#/Other#

Date	__/__/__	__/__/__
Time Completed		
Kettlebell Weight		

Conditioning notes:

Week 11, Day 2 – Strength

Bench Press, 6 sets x 3 repetitions @ 90-92% 1RM

*Work up in weight so that the final set is challenging.

Date	___/___/___	___/___/___
Weight, Set 1		
Weight, Set 2		
Weight, Set 3		
Weight, Set 4		
Weight, Set 5		
Weight, Set 6		
Total Volume		

Strength notes:

Week 11, Day 2 – Conditioning

Perform 5 sets of as many repetitions as possible of Dips. Rest 1 minute in between each set.
*For those unable to perform Dips, execute Push-ups

Date	___/___/___	___/___/___
Reps, Set 1		
Reps, Set 2		
Reps, Set 3		
Reps, Set 4		
Reps, Set 5		
Total Reps		

(5-minute Rest)

Perform 4 rounds:
Set your clock for 5 minutes, then perform 50 Double-unders; after your Double-unders, Row for as many meters as possible with the remainder of the 5 minutes. 2-minute rest in between each set.
*For those unable to perform Double-unders, execute Single-unders; for those unable to perform Single-unders, execute Jumping Jacks.

Date	___/___/___	___/___/___
Meters Rowed		

Conditioning notes:

Week 11, Day 3 – Rest

Week 11, Day 4 – Strength

Squat, 6 sets x 3 repetitions @ 90-92% 1RM
*Work up in weight so that the final set is challenging.

Date	___/___/___	___/___/___
Weight, Set 1		
Weight, Set 2		
Weight, Set 3		
Weight, Set 4		
Weight, Set 5		
Weight, Set 6		
Total Volume		

Strength notes:

Week 11, Day 4 – Conditioning

Perform as many repetitions of the following as possible in 5 rounds:

1-minute Dumbbell Snatches

1-minute Sit-ups

(30-second Rest)

Male Dumbbell weight: 35-70#/Other#

Female Dumbbell weight: 20-45#/Other#

Date	___/___/___	___/___/___
Repetitions Completed		
Dumbbell Weight		

(5-minute rest)

Perform 2 rounds of the following for time:

25 Kettlebell Deadlift High-pulls

800-meter Run

800-meter Row

*45-minute time cap.

Male Kettlebell weight: 35-70#/Other#

Female Kettlebell weight: 20-45#/Other#

Date	___/___/___	___/___/___
Time Completed		
Kettlebell Weight		

Conditioning notes:

Week 11, Day 5 – Strength

Overhead Press, 6 sets x 3 repetitions @ 90-92% 1RM
*Work up in weight so that the final set is challenging.

Date	___/___/___	___/___/___
Weight, Set 1		
Weight, Set 2		
Weight, Set 3		
Weight, Set 4		
Weight, Set 5		
Weight, Set 6		
Total Volume		

Strength notes:

Week 11, Day 5 – Conditioning

Perform as many rounds as possible in 30 minutes:

50 Push-ups

10 Box Jumps

10 Burpees

400-meter Run

Male Box height: 20-24"/Tuck Jump

Female Box height: 20"/Tuck Jump

Date	__/__/__	__/__/__
Rounds Completed		
Box Jump Height		

Conditioning notes:

Week 11, Day 6 – Run

25-minute Run for distance

Date	___ / ___ / ___	___ / ___ / ___
Distance		

Week 12, Day 1 – Strength

Deadlift, 6 sets x 3 repetitions @ 90-92% 1RM
*Work up in weight so that the final two sets are challenging.

Date	___/___/___	___/___/___
Weight, Set 1		
Weight, Set 2		
Weight, Set 3		
Weight, Set 4		
Weight, Set 5		
Weight, Set 6		
Total Volume		

Strength notes:

Week 12, Day 1 – Conditioning

10-minute, 5-repetition EMOM (every minute on the minute) Squat. At minute 0, execute 5 reps of the Squat; upon completion, rest the remainder of the minute. At minute 1, once again Squat 5 reps; upon completion, rest the remainder of the minute. Continue this process until you have completed 10 rounds. If you get to a point where you can no longer perform 5 repetitions, stop.

Male and Female Squat weight: 65% Bodyweight-Bodyweight/Other#

Date	___/___/___	___/___/___
Repetitions Completed		
Barbell Weight		

(5-minute Rest)

Perform 3 rounds:
25 Kettlebell Swings
25 Pull-ups
400-meter Run
*45-minute time cap.
**For those unable to perform Pull-ups, execute Inverted Rows.

Male Kettlebell weight: 45-70#/Other#
Female Kettlebell weight: 20-45#/Other#

Date	___/___/___	___/___/___
Time Completed		

Conditioning note:

Week 12, Day 2 – Strength

Bench Press, 6 sets x 3 repetitions @ 90-92% 1RM
*Work up in weight so that the final two sets are challenging.

Date	___/___/___	___/___/___
Weight, Set 1		
Weight, Set 2		
Weight, Set 3		
Weight, Set 4		
Weight, Set 5		
Weight, Set 6		
Total Volume		

Strength notes:

Week 12, Day 2 – Conditioning

8 Overhead Presses
8 Box Jumps
30 Sit-ups
300-meter Row
8 Overhead Presses (Add 5 pounds)
8 Box Jumps
30 Sit-ups
300-meter Row
8 Overhead Presses (Add 5 pounds)
8 Box Jumps
30 Sit-ups
300-meter Row
...and so on and so forth, until you can no longer perform 8
Overhead Presses or until you have worked out for 30 minutes.

Male Barbell starting weight begins at 50-60% of Max Press/Other#
Female Barbell starting weight begins at 30-40% of Max
Press/Other#
Male Box height: 20-24"/Tuck Jump
Female Box height: 20"/Tuck Jump

Date	___/___/___	___/___/___
Rounds Completed		
Starting Barbell Weight		
Box Jump Height		

Conditioning notes:

Week 12, Day 3 – Rest

Week 12, Day 4 – Strength

Squat, 6 sets x 3 repetitions @ 90-92% 1RM
*Work up in weight so that the final two sets are challenging.

Date	___/___/___	___/___/___
Weight, Set 1		
Weight, Set 2		
Weight, Set 3		
Weight, Set 4		
Weight, Set 5		
Weight, Set 6		
Total Volume		

Strength notes:

Week 12, Day 4 – Conditioning

Perform 3 rounds of the following:

15 Deadlifts

15 Burpees

Male Barbell weight: 185-225#/Other#

Female Barbell weight: 95-135#/Other#

Date	_____/_____/_____	_____/_____/_____
Time Completed		
Deadlift Weight		

(5-minute Rest)

2,000-meter Row

Time Completed		

Conditioning notes:

Week 12, Day 5 – Strength:

Overhead Press, 6 sets x 3 repetitions @ 90-92% 1RM
*Work up in weight so that the final two sets are challenging.

Date	__/__/__	__/__/__
Weight, Set 1		
Weight, Set 2		
Weight, Set 3		
Weight, Set 4		
Weight, Set 5		
Weight, Set 6		
Total Volume		

Strength notes:

Week 12, Day 5 – Conditioning

Perform 2 rounds of the following:
10 Dumbbell Bench Presses
10 Barbell Rows
9 Dumbbell Bench Presses
9 Barbell Rows
...and so on and so forth, until the round of 1 repetitions is complete.

Male Dumbbell weight: 45-90#/Other# (each dumbbell)
Female Dumbbell weight: 15-45#/Other# (each dumbbell)
Male Barbell weight: 40-60% Bodyweight/Other#
Female Barbell weight: 20-40% Bodyweight/Other#

Date	___/___/___	___/___/___
Time Performed		
Dumbbell Weight		
Barbell Weight		

(5-minute Rest)

Perform 8 minutes of the Farmer's Walk for distance. Every time you place the weight down, there is a 10 Depth Push-up penalty.

Male Dumbbell weight: 45-70#/Other# (each dumbbell)
Female Dumbbell weight: 20-45#/Other# (each dumbbell)

Distance Completed		

Conditioning Notes:

Week 12, Day 6 – Run

30-minute Run for distance

Date	___ / ___ / ___	___ / ___ / ___
Distance		

Week 12, Day 7 – Rest

Week 13, Day 1 – Conditioning (No Strength)

Perform for 30 minutes:
10 Dumbbell Lunges (5 per leg)
5 Dumbbell Deadlifts (same weight)
20 Sit-ups

Male Dumbbell weight: 35-70#/Other# (each dumbbell)
Female Dumbbell weight: 15-45#/Other# (each dumbbell)

Date	___/___/___	___/___/___
Rounds Completed		
Dumbbell Weight		

Conditioning notes:

Week 13, Day 2 – Conditioning (No Strength)

Perform for 30 minutes:
5 Pull-ups
15 Push-ups
25 Double-unders
*For those unable to perform Pull-ups, execute Inverted Rows.
**For those who are unable to perform Double-unders, execute Single-unders; for those who are unable to perform Single-unders, execute Jumping Jacks.

Date	___/___/___	___/___/___
Rounds Completed		

Conditioning notes:

Week 13, Day 3 – Rest

Week 13, Day 4 – Run

20-minute Run for distance

Date	___ / ___ / ___	___ / ___ / ___
Distance		

Week 13, Day 5 – Row

20-minute Row for distance

Date	___/___/___	___/___/___
Distance		

Week 13, Day 6 – Rest

Week 13, Day 7 – Rest

Week 14, Day 1 – Testing

Maximum Deadlift

Date	___ / ___ / ___	___ / ___ / ___
Weight Lifted		

Notes:

(Rest as needed)

2-minute Pull-ups
*For those unable to perform Pull-ups, execute Inverted Rows.

Date	___ / ___ / ___	___ / ___ / ___
Repetitions Completed		

Notes:

(Rest as needed)

*Continued on next page

Bodyweight Deadlifts

*Perform as many repetitions as possible; however, stop once form begins to fail, or when you are one or two reps shy of your true limit.

Date	___/___/___	___/___/___
Barbell Weight		
Repetitions Completed		

Notes:

(Rest as needed)

500-meter Row

Date	___/___/___	___/___/___
Time Completed		

Notes:

Week 14, Day 2 – Testing

Maximum Bench Press

Date	___/___/___	___/___/___
Weight Lifted		

Notes:

(Rest as needed)

800-meter Run

Date	___/___/___	___/___/___
Time Completed		

Notes:

(Rest as needed)

*Continued on next page

2-minute Push-ups

Date	___/___/___	___/___/___
Repetitions Completed		

Notes:

(Rest as needed)

7-minute Double-unders
*For those who are unable to perform Double-unders, execute Single-unders; for those who are unable to perform Single-unders, execute Jumping Jacks

Date	___/___/___	___/___/___
Repetitions Completed		

Notes:

Week 14, Day 3 – Rest

Week 14, Day 4 – Testing

Maximum Squat

Date	___/___/___	___/___/___
Weight Lifted		

Notes:

(Rest as needed)

2-minute Sit-ups

Date	___/___/___	___/___/___
Repetitions Completed		

Notes:

(Rest as needed)

*Continued on next page

Bodyweight Squats
*Perform as many repetitions as possible; however, stop once form begins to fail, or when you are one or two reps shy of your true limit.

Date	___/___/___	___/___/___
Bodyweight		
Repetitions Completed		

Notes:

(Rest as needed)

2,000-meter Row

Date	___/___/___	___/___/___
Time Completed		

Notes:

Week 14, Day 5 – Testing

Maximum Overhead Press

Date	___ / ___ / ___	___ / ___ / ___
Weight Lifted		

Notes:

(Rest as needed)

30-second Row

Date	___ / ___ / ___	___ / ___ / ___
Distance Completed		

Notes:

(Rest as needed)

*Continued on next page

7-minute Burpees

Date	___/___/___	___/___/___
Repetitions Completed		

Notes:

(Rest as needed)

2-mile Run

Date	___/___/___	___/___/___
Time Completed		

Notes:

Week 14, Day 6 – Rest

Week 14, Day 7 – Rest

CONGRATULATIONS!

We'd love to hear about your accomplishments! You can send your results to coach@farmergym.com.

Made in the USA
Coppell, TX
06 November 2020